HOW TO CURE

ACNE

How To Cure Acne

What Is Acne And The Best Treatments For Acne

Mike Rooney

TABLE OF CONTENT

The Despair Of Acne

Acne is something that most of us would experience in one time or another in our lifetime. Most of us know what it is. In fact, I don't know anyone who has never had acne.

To define acne, it is a dermatological term which includes having pimples, clogged pores and lumps or cysts on the face, chest, neck or any other part of your body. Acne is something which is most common among teenagers. However, it isn't limited to a single age group and would affect even adults in their forties.

There are many variation of this condition but none of them are life-threatening. A severe case of acne can be very problematic and leaves permanent scars on the affected areas.

Acne is generally caused because of a physical change in body tissue, or called as lesions. This is because of five changes, which includes comedos, pustule, nodule, papule and cyst. Those terms represents a range or severity of comedo at one end and cysts or nodules on the other. Comedos are generally known as blackheads and whiteheads.

Those teenagers among the ages of twelve to seventeen are most prone to this acne problem. To cure a milder situation of acne, it can be cured with over-the-counter medication. Over time, the acne goes away during their early twenties. Generally speaking, acne would affect both guys and girls equally. However, the effects on both sexes are different.

In general, young men would have a more serious, long-term form of acne. Young women, meanwhile, have a more reoccurring or irregular acne into your adulthood due to changes in your hormones or the use of cosmetics.

As we have understood briefly what acne it, we could move on to understanding it deeper and the proper treatment of it. This book discusses the different types of acne, the proper treatment and the common myths about it.

From this book, I hope the reader would have a better understanding of acne and its various types. You would learn the proper treatment and learn how to reduce the impact for those who are suffering from this condition.

This isn't a comprehensive guide for acne, but it gives the general knowledge needed and the basic knowledge on treating it. Read on to discover more.

Myths About Acne

Many problems for those who are trying to deal with acne are because of certain pervasive myths about the cause of acne. There are numerous sources of information about acne now, but there are certain myths which are being passed around to those who are unfortunately affected by this disease.

After some time, problems would be compounded. The wrong treatment based on these myths would mean a less than effective result. This does more damage if you have severe acne.

Therefore, it is very important to understand acne and the treatment types. It is important to first have a quick overview on the common myths that are out there about acne. This helps you dispel the misinformation about acne. From here, you would be able to better understand the actual cause of acne.

Myth #1: Acne Is Caused By The Wrong Diet

"Don't eat this and that, it will cause pimples!"

There are many myths about food and whether it would cause pimples. Some say that eating greasy foods would give you pimples. You would have definitely heard of this statement before. They are effectively saying that what you eat would cause acne. What this is simply untrue. This is a myth, and a very popular one on acne.

There has been extensive scientific research being done on this myth between a person's diet and the cause of acne. There has been no conclusive evidence as yet. We should realize that each of us is different and during a pimples breakout, your pimples would be worse after eating some food. This differs among different people. For example, people get a pimples breakout after eating chocolate while some would have no effect.

Some people, meanwhile, have a breakout when they drink or eat too much of coffee or seafood. It is a good example of what they should cut back. If there are certain drinks or food that is affecting your acne, you should cut back and see if it helps your pimples condition.

Myth #2: The Cause Of Acne Is Stress

Stress isn't a direct cause of acne. However, certain types of stress would cause your body to produce a certain hormone known as cortisol. This is a hormone which irritates acne.

You can take certain medication to alleviate or control your stressful situation indirectly. Besides that, it is also important to deal with emotional problems like depression as they are important factors in the acne production. However, certain medications shouldn't be taken as acne is a possible side effect. Check the labels before you take them.

Myth #3: Acne Is Because Of Poor Hygiene

This is a very common myth among many people. It doesn't matter if you scrub your face or body which is affected by acne, it doesn't affect the pimples situation that you have. As a matter of fact, this regimen of scrubbing and washing could actually aggravate your skin and make your acne situation worse.

You might have heard of this myth from the people around you from your family and friends, but the cause of acne isn't poor hygiene.

However, it doesn't mean that you shouldn't take care of your hygiene. With proper hygiene, you can reduce the acne effects, when used together with acne treatment products. Rather than frequent washing, you should wash your face with mild soap two to three times a day. After that, gently pat it dry. Don't scrub it dry.

Myth #4 Acne Would Go Away By Itself

This isn't true and you would need proper acne treatment to treat it. There are several forms of acne treatment product available today and you should take some time to find for the right one to cure your acne situation.

In most cases, visiting a dermatologist should be considered. They are able to give you the relevant advice to ensure an improvement of your condition.

Myth #5 Tanning Clears Your Skin

Tannin doesn't clear up your skin at all. However, it may have a reverse effect. It may seem like your condition is improving at first, but tanning merely masks the acne that you have.

In truth, the sun would make your skin drier and more irritable. This causes more attack of acne.

If you are doing a tan, you should make sure that you use a sunscreen which doesn't contain oils or other forms of chemicals which would clog up your pores and causes your acne condition to be worse.

Myth #6 Popping Your Pimples Help Control The Acne Situation

This may seem true but nothing is further from the truth. Popping your pimples would speed up the healing but this action would actually make the situation worse. This is because when you pop the whitehead caused the bacteria to be pushed even deeper into your skin. This means that the infection would grow even more, and lead to further scarring.

Myth #7 Only Teenagers Would Be Victims Of Acne

Trust me; this is one of the biggest myth in acne. According to research 25-35 percent of acne sufferers are those between the ages of 25 and 50. Don't just think that the acne condition is confined to teenagers.

****

I have shared these seven myths with you, but this isn't all. There are more myths out there that are circulating around the world about this acne condition. There are many more myths about acne that you would need to know.

However, this seven myths are the most important to know. The reason why you should know about these myths is so that the reader would understand better about the acne condition.

This is a very complicated because of the certain myths that are so popular. Therefore, when reading about acne, you need to be very careful of what you read and use some common sense. Don't simply believe in anything you read.

Dealing With Teenage Acne For Parents

One way or another, acne has affected us at one time or another. If you have a teenage child, you would know how difficult it is in dealing with acne. This is a very sensitive condition that would affect a child's self-image and social life. In more serious cases, it could even lead to withdrawal and depression.

In dealing with this, the parent needs to be very skillful. Tell your teenager that you are there for him or her and you are willing to help, whatever it takes. You can also share your own experiences with him or her and this would give them a wider perspective on their condition.

In may be even more difficult if they don't want to talk about it. However, you can be certain that acne is something that bothers them a lot. Your teenager may most probably be trying everything in order to control their acne situation.

As adults, we already know that acne wouldn't last forever. We know that given time and the appropriate attention, it would be cleared over time. However, most teenagers find it hard to believe because of the severity of their condition. As such, a lot of angst is in them.

It is perhaps a very difficult thing to talk about acne with your teenager. They are embarrassed by their appearance and would merely pretend that it isn't an issue for them. The most important thing in this situation is to be understanding and supportive. You should also give them all the moral support them need. Being a source of quality information and advice is also a tremendous help to curing their acne situation.

Perhaps the one effective method is to learn as much as you can about the different types of acne and how to treat them. This may sound simple, but it goes a long way in being an effective guidance for your children when confronted with decisions about their acne treatment.

You would be in a better position to help them in selecting the appropriate acne medication and determine if they should meet a dermatologist. Don't go into this trap of believing that just because you had acne as a teenager and it when away, and you have all the knowledge about it. There are more to know that that.

Various advances in scientific research on acne have unearthed new information. Besides that, there are many different medications now in the market that could help your teenager even more. They may be able to treat their condition even faster than before. When you start knowing what is available, you can subsequently find the best option for your child.

The Real Cause Of Acne

Years of research have tried to discover the real cause of acne, but no conclusive evidence has been found. Through the endless research of acne, no primary cause of acne has been found to date. Research are still being done till now.

However, through the years of research done, doctors and medical researchers have found certain risk factors that are involved and what ultimately contributes to the development of acne. To some researchers, the primary cause of it is genetics and hormones. Though, this isn't the same for everyone. There are still many other different factors.

In many instances, there are factors which create the conditions for acne's formation. These factors include certain types of cosmetics, medications and unsuitable personal hygiene.

The other main reason is also the environment you are in. People who work with certain chemicals or exposed to greases or oil have a greater probability of developing acne because those material could clog your pores, thus creating a pimples problem.

Hormones Factor

During puberty, the human body produces certain hormones which cause acne. These hormones are called as androgens or male sex hormones. This increases in every teenager, in both boys and girls. These hormones cause the over-stimulation and enlargement of the sebaceous glands which can be found in the pores of the skin or hair follicles.

This extra sebum that your sebaceous glands produce mixes with the dead skin cells and bacteria on the skin. This block the pores, the bacteria multiply and cause an inflammation. This leads to the problems associated with acne.

The most common sufferers of acne are teenagers. This is because of the shift in hormones, normally associated with puberty.

Approximately 85% of people would develop acne during the ages of 12 to 30.

Another important thing to remember is that acne can also be causes by other hormonal changes. This include during pregnancy, menstrual cycle and menopause. Besides that, when women are in the beginning or ending of their birth control usage, hormonal fluctuations could occur and causes acne in some women.

Other hormonal fluctuations in adults could also cause the production spike of sebum in the sebaceous glands. This means that acne can affect almost everyone, due to the changes or hormones.

Genetics Factor

The other main factor of acne is genetics, or heredity. Researchers have solid reason to believe that this tendency of developing acne is inherited from parents. Studies from various scientists have found the link between those who are presently suffering from acne and the presence of acne in their family history.

Still, acne isn't a disease that is inherited, at least not medically. However, acne is way more common among children whose parents have had a history of having acne. The research on the correlation between genetics and acne is still continuing. There wouldn't be a doubt that new knowledge about this condition would be known. Who knows, perhaps a deeper genetic cause may be discovered.

Other Acne Factors

Over-Abrasive Cleansing

Certain facial products which aren't suitable could dry your skin and cause your body to produce an excessive amount of sebum to compensate for this. Using harsh exfoliators could damage those spots and spread infection over your body.

Medication Inappropriate

Certain drugs would create terrible side effects, thus causing acne. Among the main medication which causes acne include lithium, steroids, anti-depressants and anti-anxiety medication.

Inappropriate Cosmetics

Certain cosmetics have ingredients which would affect the structure of your hair follicles. This would lead to an over-production of sebum. This clogs the pores, causing pimples.

Flare Up Factors

Besides the factors mentioned in the past few pages, there are also several other factors which cause the acne to flare up and create many problems for the sufferer. The factors are included in the next few pages so you better understand acne and would understand better the element and causes of this acne disorder which is so uncomfortable.

Environmental Issue

A person who works in a factory or garage would be exposed to certain chemicals. These chemicals which are present in these environments could create an acne flare-ups and lead to pimples.

For example, oils in contact with your skin over a certain period would clog up your pores or irritate the skin. Pollution has the same effect as well.

Pressure From Apparel Or Helmets

When there is a certain pressure from your apparel or helmet, or if you have a backpack pressing against your shoulder; the irritation and acne breakout potential increases. Friction from wearing tight clothing, when pressured against the body could affect your pores and cause an acne flare up.

Skin Being Scrubbed Heavily

This happens when you choose to squeeze your blackheads or whiteheads. Doing this would cause the infection to more deep into your skin. This leads to scarring over time.

Diet

For some people, diet could affect their acne. Research has proven that food has no direct correlation to the cause of acne, but certain food would definitely affect the acne condition.

Various Types of Acne

(1)Acne Vulgaris

Acne Vulgaris is the most common form of acne and what normally affects adolescents. However, without proper care, this condition may be even more severe when the sufferer reaches adulthood.

Milder form of this acne has certain characteristics, which includes:

- **Blackheads**: The blackheads would appear when your pores are partially blocked. This would allow certain trapped sebum, dead skin cells and bacteria to gradually drain to the surface. As such, the dark color normally associated with its appearance isn't because of dirt but a skin reaction of its own pigment and melanin, while it reacts with the oxygen in the air. Whiteheads have shorter life cycle, while blackheads have a firmer structure and generally takes longer to clear.

- **Whiteheads**: This results when your pore is completely blocked. Sebum, bacteria and dead skin cells are blocked and this causes a white appearance on the surface.
- **Pustules**: These are similar to whiteheads, but are slightly inflamed. It appears as a red circle with a yellow or white center. This is commonly known as 'zits'.

- **Papules**: This are inflamed red, tender bumps with no head.

The more severe form acne vulgaris are distinguished when there are cysts and nodules:

- **Nodules**: Nodular acne consists of larger spots which are very painful and could last for months. They are larger and harder bumps under the skin's surface and scarring is extremely common. Don't ever squeeze such acne as it would cause severe scarring on your skin. The lesion may last for a couple of month when you squeeze them compared to when they are left untouched.

- **Cysts**: Acne cysts have a similar appearance to nodule. However, it is often pus-filled and has a diameter of more than two inches across. It is also very painful and scarring is very common. Like nodules, don't ever squeeze them as you put a risk of inflammation or a deeper infection.

(2)Adult Acne

Acne vulgaris could also affect adults over the age of thirty. These are known as adult acne. This may be very surprising to the sufferer because they might not have the situation when they were a teenager, but they have this condition when they are adults.

This is because acne is more commonly associated with a hormonal fluctuation during the puberty period. However, adults who have them should be inspected to find out the original cause. This is especially important if one experience this condition for the first time during their adulthood.

There are several main reasons as to why acne appears after the age of thirty. They include:

- Acne that happens when a person is a teenager reappears again in adulthood. There has been no clear scientific back up as for why this happens, but it is one of the key reasons for this happening in adults.

- Women after pregnancy may have this condition where there hasn't been any activity for a certain period. This is also a case for women who are in their menstrual period.

- Acne can appear in adults who haven't had this condition before. This condition is normally because of external pollutants. If you find yourself an adult and having this condition, you should speak to a dermatologist or a doctor immediately.

These are several reasons. However, there are still other possible causes of acne in adults. This includes:

- **Constant physical pressure on skin**. This happens when one wears certain apparels or a backpack. There would be a certain pressure on your skin and this leads to breakouts over time.

- **Medication**. Certain medications induce acne. These include anabolic steroids, anti-tuberculosis drugs rifampin, lithium and other medications that have iodine in them.

- **Metabolic changes**. Hormonal changes like during an adult are pregnant or during the menstruation period produces acne in adults.

- **Certain industrial chemicals**. In some types of industrial environment creates acne-like symptoms. Chloracne, a form of skin disorder can also be caused. This condition is caused by an over-exposure to chemicals like chlorinated dioxins. This is a very serious condition.

(3)Rosacea

Rosacea is diagnosed as acne, but it is in fact, not acne. Rosacea affects a great deal of people in the United States, mostly when the sufferer is above the age of thirty. It normally appears as red rash on the nose, forehead, cheeks and chin.

It is accompanied by pimples, bumps and skin blemishes. The similarities of symptoms make it why it is often mistaken for acne. Besides, this redness also make the blood vessels becomes more visible on the skin.

This condition is more prevalent in women compared to men. However, if this condition happens to men, it would be more severe. When seeking treatment for rosacea, you need to realize that the treatments are very different compared to common acne.

(4)Acne Mechanica

Acne Mechanica is caused by external mechanical forces. This includes constant pressure or friction, covered skin and heat. Those who are involved in certain sports, military or certain high-activity jobs are most prone to this. This is nothing new where restrictive clothing or tight-fitting clothes are worn for an extended period of time.

These jobs may also include factory work where the employee is busy with certain repetitive tasks that would irritate the skin and lead to break outs. Soldiers who wear uniforms most of the time or carry backpacks which hurt the skin can create an acne issue.

Not only do what they wear affect their acne condition, but because of the extreme temperature that they find themselves in, it could further complicate the acne condition. This leads to inflammation and further breakouts over time.

Other possible causes of this acne condition also include:

- **Bra straps** which fit uncomfortably on the skin
- **Head bands** which are worn that rubs on the forehead and makes the skin irritable
- **Physical contact with musical instrument**, creates fiction over a certain period
- **Wearing tight clothing**, this include jeans or certain undergarments that would make your skin uncomfortable

(5)Acne Cosmetica

Women who are always wearing make-up or certain cosmetics may find that they have acne on their cheeks or forehead. This condition is known as acne cosmetica and is caused by the cosmetics that are being used. There are several forms of cosmetics.

Pomade Acne

This condition happens when a person adapt to a new hair style. When hairstyle trends change, it is very common for the younger generation to change with them. They may need a certain cosmetic called pomade to style their hair. Pomade is used when a hairstyle requires curly hair to be straightened or molded into certain shapes.

The setback of using pomade is a pomade acne attack. This acne happens on the scalp of your head, temples or forehead. Any place that pomade makes contact with your skin, there is a potential of pomade.

Almost all pomades are considered in the pore clogging cosmetics category. Heavy oils used in pomades could clog your skin and this result in the formation of comedones. Additionally, certain chemicals in this substance would irritate the skin and contribute to inflammation.

Excoriated Acne

Excoriated means the scratching or abrading the skin. Excoriated acne is caused by such scratching or other physical contact. This form of acne is defined by the sufferer's behavior

When the sufferer keeps on picking and scraping every single pimple and blemish on their skin, they are said to have an excoriated acne condition.

Deep irritation and scarring can result from this excessive physical touch on the sufferer's skin. While it may appear as a mild form of acne which has no nodules or pustules, this condition may be intolerable to the sufferer.

There is an almost psychological urge to remove their skin lesions or blemish. This urge can be very damaging and a dermatologist should be consulted to seek the right treatment.

Infantile Acne

Infantile acne is a condition that occurs in certain newborns. It occurs mainly on your nose and cheeks and caused by certain hormonal changes that occurs while your fetus is developing in the womb. This form of acne clears up without treatment in a few weeks.

However, those who suffer from infantile acne have certain aspect that need to be considered. You can start by trying to cleanse it with mild soap and water.

If this doesn't help clear the acne, then use a mild topical agent such as benzoyl peroxide for infants. This helps the current situation and prevents scarring over the long term. If this still doesn't help, seek the help of a dermatologist.

Important Factors To Consider When Your Child Has Acne

- **Early Hormonal Production**: There is a huge possibility that the infant has a condition which causes the production of sexual hormones early in their lifetime. This is especially in the production of androgen which is linked to the acne problem. If such, seek medical help to avoid further complication with the child's development.

- **Growth And Development Anomalies**: When having acne in such an early stage in a child's life, it is an indication of development problems that would only show up until later in life. As such, a pediatrician should be consulted to decide if this is a possibility. The pediatrician is able to determine better the condition you child is facing.

- **Family History**: Without a doubt, genetics is a key factor in acne development in infants. Check if the child's parents or siblings have had severe acne in the past or even currently.

- **Drug Induced Acne**: When exposed to certain form of medication, the child would get acne or acneiform lesions. This medication may include corticosteroids or iodine.

Dealing With Severe Acne

Many dermatologists recognize a minimum of four kinds of acne as severe. This is based on both the types of lesions that the acne produces on the body together with the long term effects the acne could have on the sufferer.

This severe condition affects more than the body. It could also affect every single aspect of a person's life, from physical to psychological. It is very painful and heartbreaking when it comes to dealing with disfiguring form of acne.

Teenagers who have severe acne have the tendency to create emotional scars which last a long period.

This severely lowers the quality of life and destroys self-esteem over the longer term. In this chapter, we would learn all about the severe forms of acne. By the end of this chapter, you are better equipped to determine if you are really having severe acne and whether you need to take further action. It covers all four types of severe acne.

(1)Acne conglobata

The most severe form of acne vulgaris is acne conglobate.

This is a very serious consideration which is characterized by interconnected large and numerous nodules, along with widespread blackheads. As these lesions become ulcerated, they would cause irrevocable damage to the skin. This condition is found most common on your face, back, chest, buttocks, thighs and upper arms.

The people who normally have this condition are normally in the age group of eighteen to thirty years. It is more probable for men to get this condition compared to women.

This condition also persists over a few years, lying dormant until certain conditions causes it to reappear. Like all kinds of acne problems, the cause of this condition is still unknown.

(2)Acne Fulminans

This form of acne is a sudden form of acne conglobate which normally affects young men. There are several symptoms of this condition which includes ulcerating acne.

Like most common form of acne conglobate, lesions would cover large portion of the facial region and extremities. Over time, disfiguring scars would eventually develop.

Acne fulminans is unique in a sense that it includes aches on your joints on your knees and hips. Besides that you may also have fever symptoms and sudden weight loss. However, these symptoms depend on the individual.

(3)Gram-negative folliculitis

The third type of severe acne is Gram-Negative Folliculitis. It is a form of acne which happens by an inflammation of your follicles caused by a bacterial infection. It is characterized by cysts and pustules. Some research has found that this disorder can be caused by complications from long term antibiotic treatment of acne vulgaris.

This condition is called "gram-negative" because gram is a form of blue stain used in laboratory testing for microscopic organism. Therefore, bacteria which doesn't stain blue are known as "gram-negative". Similar to many form of extreme acne, this condition is very rare and very few researches have conclusive evidence about the cause of this condition.

(4)Pyoderma Faciale

This form of severe acne is something that affects only females between 20 and 40 years of age.

Those who suffer from this extreme condition have large painful nodules, pustules and certain sores that would leave scarring over a certain period. It form abruptly and this condition would normally occur on woman's skin who haven't have acne before.

This form of acne is only on your face and it doesn't last for longer than a year. But, it could cause a lot of problems in just a short period of time.

Natural Remedies For Acne

It is something of a controversial topic when it comes to the use of natural remedies to cure any form of medical situation. It is hard to separate those natural remedies which are effective compared to the myths which are being brought about by years of tradition.

It would be foolish for anyone to just push aside the benefits of natural remedies without even trying it. Natural remedies are extremely powerful and most of them are just pure common sense.

Herbs not only help cure your medical conditions but also help regain a sense of health. Natural remedies are also incredibly successful in dealing with certain mild cases of acne. However, if you situation become severe, you must definitely seek a dermatologist or qualified physician.

For many centuries, human civilization has been relying solely on herbal and natural remedies to treat many ailments. To find a method of curing sickness, a person needs to go into the woods to search natural treatment of curing acne. Nature provided the needs through various herbal methods that have great medicinal value.

There aren't online stores where you can get your prescription for medications or doctor who could provide you with the required medication. The earliest doctors were herbalists who depend solely on the power of natural herbs for cure.

Natural remedies which are discovered by ancient herbalist are the basis of scientists who discover other form of medication. They created synthetic substitutes for such herbs and create another form of medication. Therefore, it could be said that natural remedies are the basis of all forms of medication.

Common Natural Remedies

Using Hot Or Cold Compresses - This is a very important remedy used for many centuries. It may seem simple - using a hot and cold wet towel - but it is incredibly effective. It helps reduce swelling and eliminate pores which are clogged. This is a major reason for acne. Using hot or cold compresses helps in dealing with acne.

Oils And Juices - It may seem very strange that natural substances can help with removing acne scars. Using almond oil would help this purpose. To alleviate cysts presence, apricot juice would help. Simply place them on your skin.

Citric fruit juices, like lemon juice, serve as a great natural exfoliate. It would help remove the dead skin cells which cause the pores to clog. Simply place it on the face for around ten minutes and then rinse it with cold water.

Drink A Lot Of Water - This is perhaps the simplest natural remedy tip, but perhaps it's the most important. The idea behind it is that if you drink enough water a day, your body is cleanse enough to remove the toxic which contributes to the spread of acne in your body. The ideal number of glasses of water to drink daily is 8 glasses.

You should also realize that some natural herbalist don't just recommend drinking plain ordinary water but also recommend adding herbal ingredients like corn or fenugreek seeds.

Simply mix these herbal ingredients into the water and boil them, as simple as that.

Fenugreek Leaves - This is a form of remedy that provides prevention of potential breakouts. The process includes taking the fenugreek leaves and crushing them, while making a paste out of it. Apply the paste onto the infected areas each night. From there, wash it away the next morning with warm water.

Distilled White Vinegar - This is a form of topical solution. Simply let the vinegar sit on the infected area for around ten minutes. From there, rinse it carefully with cool water. Very often, the vinegar is too strong and therefore you should dilute it with water. However, make sure it is not over-diluted as it would defeat the purpose.

Honey Mask - Honey is actually a very powerful chemical substance. Honey has anti-bacterial qualities that are applied on your face and helps kill surface bacteria. This should be applied around one of two times each week. If the results are great, continue doing it. If not, stop. This natural remedy may not suit everyone.

Reduce The Use Of Cosmetics - This isn't a natural remedy, but just pure common sense. Many teenage girls are guilty of using cosmetics. Be aware that chemicals from cosmetics are incredibly harmful. As such, stop using it right away if you have an acne situation. These cosmetics would clog your pores and lead to pimple breakouts.

Further Natural Remedies

Besides these common natural remedies for acne, there are several other forms of remedies that are available and effective. Among them include:

Vitamin A - Vitamin A, when used in the right quantity, is able to treat severe forms of acne. However, it should be clear that you must consult a physician first. Over-dosage of Vitamin A can be very toxic. Ask your physician for the right dosage.

Diet and supplements - In this current day and age, most of our food have pesticides and fertilizers. This has taken a toll on the nutrient content of the food that we eat. It's unlike last time where the food we eat comes from the ground, without any of these chemicals. Besides that, our food has other chemical preservatives that are very harmful and be a cause of certain acne breakouts.

To fight this, start taking a more balanced diet and eat some supplements. This would go a long way to prevent certain chemical conditions and ensure that your acne condition doesn't become worst.

Echinacea and Oregon grape - These two herbs are extremely useful in boosting your immune system and combat different factors of acne bacteria. Over time, the use of this herb wouldn't just cure your acne situation but also improve your overall health.

Zinc - When Zinc is added into your diet, this helps aid the healing of acne and prevent scarring on your body or face.

Over-the-Counter Acne Remedies

When it comes to over-the-counter treatment for acne, there are many types that you can use. People who have acne normally go to local pharmacy and get some over-the-counter medication purely base on the recommendations of their friends or which one they see from television advertisement.

However, despite the good intention of your close ones, it is always a good idea to get advice from a physician first before using any such medication. The doctor or dermatologist would be able to provide you the best advice and give you additional suggestions based on your current situation.

If you go to any pharmacy, you would see a large selection of acne treatment products and would be very difficult to choose the right one. Don't depend on the recommendation of your close ones.

Yes, they might have used a certain medications and fix their acne problem, but it doesn't mean that it fits everyone. What works for a person doesn't work for everyone. Besides that, there is a possibility that certain ingredients in the acne medication may not suit you.

Benzoyl peroxide is one of the main ingredients in acne medication. This is typically found in certain ointments or gels. The purpose of this ingredient is that it helps to combat the bacteria that would cause acne. It also helps in removing dead skin cells which accumulates on your skin's surface.

Note that dead skin cells, when combined with sebum, create whiteheads and blackhead. This ingredient has been proven safe and effective in dealing with lesions. It is also an ingredient that helps with the prevention of acne once a breakout is cleared by ensuring that the skin is free from acne-causing bacteria. The possible side effect from this is dry skin. However, this could be easily avoided by reducing the frequency of use.

Another main ingredient found in most acne medications is salicylic acid. The role of this ingredient is that it helps prevent acne by clearing up the dead skin cells that accumulate too quickly and clogs the pores. If your skin has cleared up and your medication contains this ingredient, it is recommended to use this as it helps prevent future outbreaks of acne. However, using this ingredient has side effects as well: You may have dry, irritated skin.

Other Ingredients In OTC Medications

Besides these common ones, you have to know of the other types of ingredients you may see in your acne medication like sulphur and resorcinol.

Resorcinol is an ingredient which causes the top layer of your skin to peel. This means that your dead skin cells which clog the pores would peel as well. It is generally combined with sulphur to be more effective. Although it is hard to understand how sulphur would be able to affect your acne condition, it has been used effectively for many years.

Besides that, sulphur is also known to be combined with other ingredients like salicylic acid and benzoyl peroxide.

Among all the ingredients mentioned on dealing with acne or preventing an outbreak, the most versatile is probably benzoyl peroxide as it could be used in cleansing liquids or bars. They are also used in other skin products like lotion, gels and cream.

Generally speaking, cleansing products should be used around once or twice a day while creams and lotions are used as and when you need them. To ensure effectiveness, they should be applied on the skin around the acne together with the pimples themselves. Avoid contact with your eyes as it would be irritating and cause inflammation.

Prescriptions For Acne

Milder or moderate form of acne could be easily treated with over-the-counter medications. However, when dealing with more severe acne, the only alternative is to seek the right treatment from a dermatologist. In such cases, the doctor would recommend prescription medication to deal with the severe acne condition.

Such medications could be even more effective in dealing with moderate acne that normal over-the-counter treatment. Generally speaking, there are two types of prescription medication for acne - oral and topical.

Antibiotics

Antibiotics are used commonly in fighting acne and can be taken orally or in lotion form. Topical prescription medication would include certain ingredients like retinoid or zinc. When treating antibiotic, the most common prescription is tetracycline and it is used in killing the bacteria responsible for acne. It also reduces inflammation.

This treatment would take several weeks or months in order to be effective. Even after the acne has cleared up, it is very important to continue using antibiotics to ensure full cure.

It should be noted that tetracycline has certain side effects. When the patient is exposed to sun lights for too long, bad sunburns would happen. Other side effects also include dizziness, hives and an upset stomach. Women taking tetracycline would also be susceptible to an increase in vaginal yeast incidences.

Ointments And Topical Solutions

In general, there are fewer complications when using antibiotic ointments compared to oral antibiotics.

Similarly to oral antibiotics, topical treatments are very effective in killing bacteria which causes acne. If you use ointments with other topical treatments like benzoyl peroxide, the bacteria would be able to develop resistance to antibiotics. From here, it would increase the level of prevention that you experience.

Retinoid

Retinoid is an acne medication which is derived from Vitamin A. It is applied directly on the skin in the form of creams or lotions. Topical retinoid medications are very useful in the treatment of blackheads and whiteheads by opening up the clogged pores.

Oral retinoid, meanwhile, are used to treat the more severe acne problems. They have a greater probability of dealing with lesions and breakouts which don't respond to other form of treatment. It causes the upper layer of the skin to peel and thus open the pores. It also ensures that your body produces sebum. Sebum is the substances which causes oily skin.

Like many types of prescription medication which are strong, there are a number of side effects which are extremely serious when using oral retinoids. It could cause liver damage and depression.

As such, you need to ensure that you have the medical attention of a professional doctor. This is to ensure that you aren't affected adversely by this form of treatment. It could also cause birth defects on the baby if pregnant mothers take them while pregnant. As such, you should be very careful about the use. Women should consult their doctor if they want to take this.

Birth Control Pills

It might be very surprising to you, but birth control pills are known to be incredibly effective in treating acne in women. This is because this substance changes the hormone levels in your body. It reduces the testosterone level in your body, which is the cause of acne problem.

Surgery

Surgery is only considered when every form of medicinal treatment is tried. Those who have a history of persistent acne problems would seek many different methods. After meeting a dermatologist, he or she may advise you on considering surgery. This includes laser therapy or acne surgery.

If you are considering using any form of surgery, you should take time to consider the surgical processes. This would include the number of treatments required, potential side effects from treatment and the consequent costs.

Besides that, it is also very important that you choose a process which is used to reduce the cause of acne, not just the effects (which are the scarring).

Acne Surgery

When it comes to acne surgery, the process is to make an incision into the affected area and gradually draining the clogged area. Process for whiteheads or blackheads wouldn't involve surgery but it is done by an esthetician, dermatologist or nurse. It is done by a small, pointed blade. They would first open the comedones and slowly remove the material using a comedones extractor.

With this procedure of excisional surgery, severe cysts could be drained and removed easily. This procedure has to be done in a sterile environment. This is to ensure that the risk of bacterial infection spreading is minimal. Please also remember that this procedure should only be done by a trained professional. Note that if cysts aren't extracted carefully, a serious infection can happen and create subsequent scarring.

Forms of Physical Treatment

There are three common forms of physical treatment when dealing with acne. They are:

- **Comedo Extraction**. In this procedure, you simply apply anesthetic cream to the immediate area of a breakout. From here, the comedones are extracted using an instrument which is like a pen.

  It opens the top gently to allow the gradual removal of dead skin cells and sebum from follicle. After this, antibiotic cream is normally applied.

- **Exfoliation**. This treatment is the process of removing the top later of the skin. This is done using either chemicals or certain sort of abrasive. Using chemicals, it is done with salicylic or glycolic acid. It works by destroying a tiny microscopic layer of the skin cells to unclog the pores and remove the dead cells from building up. using an abrasive cloth or liquid scrub can also achieve the same aim.

- **Drainage**. With certain form of severe acne, the cysts could form under the skin and be very painful. It could even disfigure your face. To treat these smaller cysts, use cortisone injections and they would flatten the lesions for a few days.

  However, to treat larger cysts, the best alternative is to drain them and then surgically remove them.

  This process of draining could easily relieve the pain associated with cysts and reduce the chances of scarring. It is very important to not to try and drain the cysts by yourself.

This could create an infection, which lead to further scarring. Find a professional to help you with it.

Laser Treatment

The treatments using laser simply involve using the various wavelengths to aim directly at the affected area of your skin. The wavelengths would pulsate on the skin and destroy any overly-huge sebaceous glands and acne lesions.

Through laser treatment, the damaged outer layers of the skin can be removed and this initiates the growth of new cells. The intensity of the laser is dependent on the laser technician. He would decide on it based on the necessity.

Laser therapy has many benefits. However, there still isn't conclusive research done to prove the effectiveness on a while. There are certain debates going on about this issue.

Although it has shown to be effective in improving your skin's appearance, there are certain side effects.

One of the most common side effects is that the patient would experience a red, burned skin after this treatment which could last for a few weeks. Those who have a darker color of skin could end up having skin discoloration after laser treatment. The skin's appearance could be uneven if laser isn't used in a right way.

Prevent Acne Before It Becomes A Problem

Acne can be a huge problem. It can create harm not only physically but psychologically. Anyone who has experienced it, or know of anyone who has this condition would know how demoralizing it is. As such, it is better to first look to prevent it before it becomes a problem over the long term.

Here is a general checklist for preventing acne problems:

- **Avoid Alcohol** - This isn't just alcoholic drinks. Don't use certain products like toners on your skin too. They contain a very heavy concentration of isopropyl alcohol and does more damage than good.

- **Don't Wash Your Face Too Much** - Many people believe in the myth that dirt is the cause of acne, but this is simply not true. Many times, the reason they have this condition is that they over wash their face. Limit it to twice a day and you would reduce the risk of increasing the breakouts.

- **Stick To The Right Regimen** - Find the right treatment and medication method. Don't move away from it unless you achieve results or if you find the condition getting worse.

- **Use Skin Products Carefully** - You should choose the skin products you use properly. Don't get those harsh or abrasive scrubs that would tear the skin and aggravate the acne condition.

- **Clean After Exercise** - After a workout, look to clean yourself well. The clothes that you wear during sports can be an acne problem. The friction and moisture from the clothes create a condition for acne production.

- **Don't Touch Or Pick On Your Face** - This is common sense. Your hands are full of bacterial infection. These would go into the pores and create an acne situation.

Resource 1 - Acne No More!

Medical Researcher, Nutritionist, Health Consultant and Former Acne Sufferer Teaches You How To:

- **Permanently Cure Your Acne Within 2 Months**
- End The Breakouts & See Results In Less Than 7 Days!
- **Eliminate Blackheads, Excessive Oiliness and Redness**
- Remove Most Types of Scars and Acne Marks
- **Look Better, Feel Better and Regain Your Self Esteem**
- Improve The Quality Of Your Life Dramatically!
- **Step-By-Step Fully Illustrated Guides**

Discover How He's Cured Himself From Severe Acne and Taught Thousands of People Worldwide to Get The Clearest Skin They Ever Had

http://acnenomore.wellbeingvalley.com/

Resource 2 - Cure Acne In 14 Days

This resource is a tremendous resource for those who want to only use natural forms of treatment. In just 14 Days, this guide promises to:

- **Gets rid of those tender red bumps**
- **Gets rid of blackheads**
- **Gets rid of whiteheads**
- **Gets rid of pimples**
- **Gets rid of zits**

Using only **ALL-NATURAL**

cures!

Go to this link to find out more:

http://acnecure.wellbeingvalley.com/

www.ingramcontent.com/pod-product-compliance
Lightning Source LLC
Chambersburg PA
CBHW070552290526
45790CB00002B/662